The Ultimate Cookbook to Boost Testosterone levels

Best Recipes That Are Proven to Increase Testosterone

BY: Allie Allen

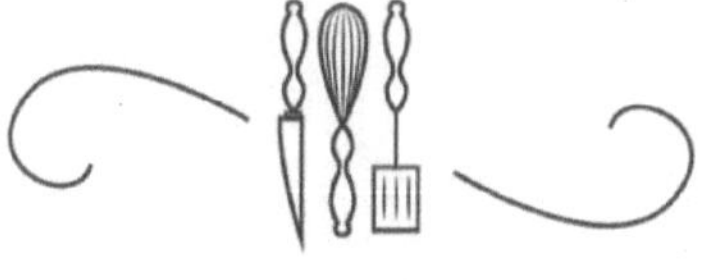

COOK & ENJOY

Copyright 2019 Allie Allen

Copyright Notes

Table of Contents

Testosterone Boosting Recipes

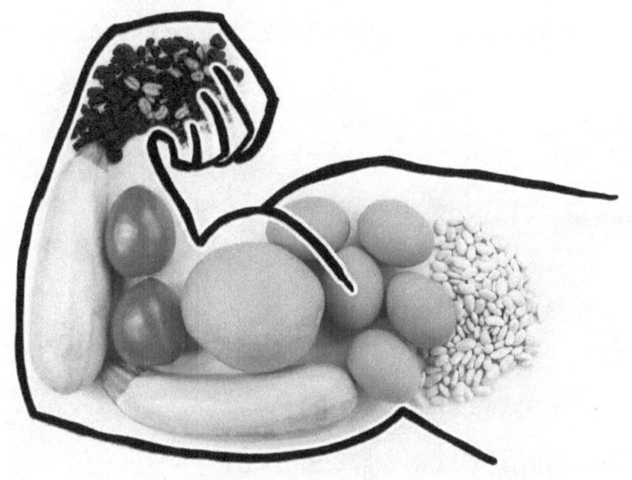

ssssssssssssssssssssssssssssssssssssssssssssssssssss

1) Spinach Stuffed Chicken Breasts

Spinach, chicken and garlic that are all used in this dish are great for boosting that 'T'. Boosting never tasted so good.

Yield: 4

Cooking Time: 85 minutes

List of Ingredients:

- Mayonnaise (½ cup)
- Garlic (2 cloves, chopped)
- Spinach (10 oz., chopped)
- Chicken breasts (4 halves, boneless and skin removed)
- Feta cheese (½ cup, crumbled)
- Bacon (4 slices)
- Salt
- Black pepper
- Mixed herb seasoning

sssssssssssssssssssssssssssssssssssssssssssssssssssssssss

Procedure:

1. Set oven to 375°F.

2. Combine garlic, mayonnaise, cheese and spinach in a bowl.

3. Use herb seasoning, black pepper and salt to season chicken. Make a slice in chicken breasts to make a pocket.

4. Use spinach blend to fill pocket and use a strip of bacon to wrap each chicken breast. Use a toothpick to hold in place.

5. Place onto baking sheet and use foil to cover. Bake for 60 minutes or until fully cooked.

6. Take from oven, remove toothpicks and serve with preferred side dish.

2) Oyster and Spinach Chowder

Oysters are filled with zinc which increases testosterone levels and also aid in muscle growth. This chowder could certainly come in handy for those cold winter nights.

Yield: 12

Cooking Time: 40 minutes

List of Ingredients:

- Olive oil (1 tbsp.)
- Milk (5 cups)
- Onion (1, chopped)
- Flour (½ cup)
- Green onions (2, sliced)
- Chicken broth (2 cups)
- Mushrooms (1 cup, sliced)
- Oysters (24 oz., canned, whole)
- Spinach (1 bunch, baby)
- Cheddar cheese (1 cup, shredded)

SSSSSSSSSSSSSSSSSSSSSSSSSSSSSSSSSSSSSSSSSSSSSSSSSSSSSSSS

Procedure:

1. Heat oil in saucepan and add green onion, mushrooms and onion; sauté until tender then add spinach a little at a time.

2. Combine 2 cups of milk and flour and put into saucepan. Add broth and leftover milk to mixture and cook until it starts to get thick. Add cheese and oysters and cook till cheese melts.

3. Serve and enjoy!

3) Quick Chili

This chili is quickly made from beans and ground beef and takes less than an hour to put together. Beef and beans both have testosterone boosting qualities.

Yield: 8

Cooking Time: 40 minutes

List of Ingredients:

- Ground beef (2 lbs.)
- Canned pinto beans (15 oz.)
- Onion (1, diced)
- Chili powder (2 tbsp.)
- Garlic (3 cloves, diced)
- Cumin (1 tbsp.)
- Canned tomatoes (29 oz., Italian style)
- White sugar (2 tbsp.)
- Salt (1 tbsp.)
- Tomato sauce (8 oz., can)
- Black pepper (1 tsp.)
- Water (1 cup)

- Hot sauce (1 tbsp.)
- Kidney beans (15 oz. can)

sssssssssssssssssssssssssssssssssssssssssssssssssssssss

Procedure:

1. Heat a large pot and cook beef until browned. Drain excess oil if necessary.

2. Put in garlic and onion and cook for 3 minutes then add all leftover ingredients.

3. Stir to combine, cover and cook for 30 minutes.

4. Serve and enjoy!

4) Slow Cooker Swiss Steak

This simple dish will be ready and waiting for you as you get home. Just set your slow cooker for 6-8 hours and come home to mouthwatering, tender steaks that will give you that testosterone kick you are looking for.

Yield: 3

Cooking Time: 6-8 hours

List of Ingredients:

- Beef blade steaks (6)
- Onion (1, sliced)
- Cayenne pepper (1 ½ tsp.)
- Dry sherry (¼ cup)
- Olive oil (4 tbsp.)
- Parsley (2 tbsp., chopped)
- Mushrooms (8 oz., white button, sliced)
- Thyme (1 tbsp., chopped)
- Beef stock (¾ cup)
- Sorghum flour (¼ cup)
- Heavy cream (½ cup)

- Salt

- Black pepper

ssssssssssssssssssssssssssssssssssssssssssssssss

Procedure:

1. Heat skillet and add oil then sauté mushrooms until golden, transfer to slow cooker.

2. Use pepper and salt to season beef and add to with a tbsp. of oil and cook until browned then put aside on a plate.

3. Add leftover oil to pan and heat then put in cayenne pepper and onion and cook for a minute then add flour and sherry; mix to combine and transfer to slow cooker.

4. Place steaks into mixture in slow cooker, set on low and cook, covered for 6-8 hours.

5. Remove steak from sauce after 8 hours and place in a covered container.

6. Add parsley and cream to sauce, stir and cook for 10 minutes.

7. Serve steaks with sauce and mashed potatoes. Enjoy!

5) Coconut Pancakes

Pancakes are usually made from flour which contains grains which decreases the levels of testosterone. These pancakes are delicious, fluffy and grain free. Coconut flour acts as a testosterone booster.

Yield: 2-3

Cooking Time: 15 minutes

List of Ingredients:

- Eggs (4)
- Vanilla (2 tsp.)
- Coconut flour (½ cup)
- Sea salt (½ tsp.)
- Milk (1 cup)
- Honey (1 tbsp.)
- Baking soda (1 tsp.)
- Coconut oil (1 tsp.)

sssssssssssssssssssssssssssssssssssssssssssssssssssssss

Procedure:

1. Heat griddle over a medium flame. Put eggs in a bowl and beat then add milk, honey and vanilla and combine.

2. Combine flour, salt and baking soda in another bowl and slowly add to wet mixture. Stir to combine until smooth.

3. Use oil to grease griddle and pour pancake batter onto griddle. Cook for 3 minutes on each side until set.

4. Top with butter, syrup and any other topping you prefer.

5. Serve and enjoy!

6) Sweet and Spicy Pumpkin Seeds

Pumpkin seeds have always been good for the prostrate and its properties are also great for boosting testosterone. Preparing pumpkin seeds is really quite simple.

Yield: 8

Cooking Time: 55 minutes

List of Ingredients:

- Pumpkin seeds (2 cups, washed and dried)
- Worcestershire sauce (1 tbsp.)
- Butter (2 tbsp., melted)
- Brown sugar (1 tbsp.)
- Salt (1 tsp.)
- Hot sauce

SSSSSSSSSSSSSSSSSSSSSSSSSSSSSSSSSSSSSSSSSSSSSSSSSSSS

Procedure:

1. Set oven to 300°F. Use foil to line a baking sheet.

2. Combine butter and pumpkin in a bowl along with all left over ingredients then place on baking sheet.

3. Bake for 45 minutes until crisp.

7) Cabbage and Eggs Scramble

The best time to start upping your testosterone levels is at breakfast with this protein filled egg and cabbage scramble. It is filling and will give you a boost not only in hormones but in your energy.

Yield: 1

Cooking Time: 10 minutes

List of Ingredients:

- Bacon (1 strip, chopped, nitrate free)
- Cabbage (2 cups, shredded)
- Eggs (2, beaten)
- Black pepper
- Seas salt

sssssssssssssssssssssssssssssssssssssssssssssssssssssss

Procedure:

1. Heat a cast iron or thick pan and add bacon to pot; cook for 3 minutes until fat is released.

2. Add cabbage to bacon and cook for 1 minute then add eggs and scramble.

3. Season with pepper and salt to taste.

4. Serve right away!

8) Rosemary Flank Steak with Fig Salsa

Sweet boosting figs complement succulent flank steak for an all-out scrumptious pair that will help improve your 'T' count.

Yield: 6

Cooking Time:

List of Ingredients:

- Garlic (2 cloves, diced)
- Black pepper (½ tsp.)
- Flank steak (1 ¼ lbs.)
- Figs (3 cups, chopped)
- Parsley (2 tbsp., chopped)
- Gorgonzola cheese (3 oz., crumbled)
- Rosemary (1 tbsp., chopped)
- Kosher salt (¾ tsp.)
- Olive oil (3 tbsp.)
- Green onion (1, diced)
- Rice wine vinegar (2 tbsp., seasoned)

Procedure:

1. Combine rosemary, salt, garlic, black pepper and a tbsp. of oil then use mixture to coat steak and let it marinate for 30 minutes in refrigerator.

2. Set grill to 400°F. Combine figs, leftover oil, green onion, vinegar and parsley. Add pepper and salt to taste.

3. Place steak on grill and cook for 5 minutes on each side or until grilled to preference. Remove from grill and put aside for 5 minutes.

4. Slice and serve and top with fig mixture and cheese.

9) He-hormone Stew

This stew is bold and is made from lamb which is rich in carnitine and zinc along with lots of celery which helps to increase androsterone which comes from testosterone. This hormone makes men seem more appealing to women and can even help to increase libido.

Yield: 2

Cooking Time: 2 hours 20 minutes (excluding marinating time)

List of Ingredients:

- Lamb Shoulder (1 ½ lbs., cubed)
- Ghee (2 tbsp.)
- Garlic (3 cloves, crushed)
- Bay leaf (1)
- Chickpeas (12 oz., cooked)
- Carrot (1, chopped)
- Black pepper
- Red wine (2 cups)
- Tomato paste (1 tbsp.)
- Onion (1, chopped)

- Celery (6 ribs, chopped)

- Potato (1, skin removed and chopped)

- Beef stock (2 cups)

- Salt

ssssssssssssssssssssssssssssssssssssssssssssssssssssssss

Procedure:

1. Place lamb into a container and pour wine onto meat. Cover and refrigerate overnight.

2. Take meat from fridge and pat with hand towels.

3. Heat a tbsp. of oil in a skillet and cook lamb for 3-5 minutes until browned all over; add pepper and salt to taste.

4. Put leftover in a large pot and heat then add garlic, tomato paste and onions and cook for a few minutes then transfer lamb to pot.

5. Use a cup of stock to deglaze skillet and add liquid to pot along with leftover stock.

6. Put in bay leaf and cover pot slightly. Cook for 90 minutes over a low flame, add water if necessary and adjust salt and pepper as desired.

7. Put in all leftover ingredients and cook for 30-45 minutes more or until meat is tender.

8. Serve and enjoy!

10) Marinated Fig Salad

Figs have been said to be an aphrodisiac and are an excellent source of zinc, magnesium, potassium and iron.

Yield: 4

Cooking Time: 45 minutes

List of Ingredients:

- Olive oil (¼ cup, extra-virgin)
- Honey (1 tbsp.)
- Figs (16, cut in halves)
- Serrano ham (4 oz., sliced)
- Balsamic vinegar (3 tbsp.)
- Dijon mustard (1 tsp., coarse)
- Mozzarella slices (8 oz.)
- Arugula (2 cups)

ssssssssssssssssssssssssssssssssssssssssssssssssssssssss

Procedure:

1. Put oil, honey, vinegar and mustard into a bowl and whisk together then add figs and set aside to marinade for 30 minutes.

2. Place arugula, ham and cheese on plate and top with marinated figs then add pepper and salt to taste.

3. Serve and enjoy!

11) Avocado Devilled Eggs with Bacon

Eggs contain aspartic acid which prompts the production of testosterone along with avocado which helps increase libido. This healthy snack can be made ahead and eaten as you desire and they are yummy.

Yield: 8-12

Cooking Time: 15 minutes

List of Ingredients:

- Avocados (2)
- Paprika (1 tsp.)
- Olive oil (1 tbsp.)
- Mustard (1 tsp.)
- Eggs (12, hard boiled)
- Bacon (6-8 slices)
- Lemon juice (1 tsp.)
- Garlic (1 clove, crushed)

sssssssssssssssssssssssssssssssssssssssssssssssssssss

Procedure:

1. Slice eggs in half and take out yolks and put into a bowl.

2. Heat skillet and cook bacon until crisp, remove from pot and place onto paper towels to remove excess oil.

3. Add leftover ingredients to egg yolks and combine until creamy.

4. Spoon mixture into egg whites and crumble bacon and top eggs.

5. Add a dash of paprika to eggs and serve. Leftovers should be stored in a covered container in refrigerator.

12) Breaded Turkey Breasts

Turkey has more protein than chicken which is of course an advantage in helping to increase your testosterone. The added protein will also help you build muscle and strong bones. Be careful not to overcook the turkey breasts.

Yield: 4

Cooking Time: 45 minutes

List of Ingredients:

- Bread crumbs (1 cup)
- Milk (1 cup)
- Parmesan cheese (¼ cup, grated)
- Turkey breast (1 lb., boneless)
- Italian seasoning mix (2 tsp.)
- Olive oil (¼ cup)
- Salt
- Black pepper

ssssssssssssssssssssssssssssssssssssssssssssssssssssss

Procedure:

1. Combine cheese, seasoning and crumbs in a bowl. Put milk into another bowl. Dip meat into milk and roll in dry mix.

2. Heat skillet and add oil then cook for 4-5 minutes in each side.

3. Take from heat, serve with desired side and enjoy!

13) Testo Burger

Bacon and beef are excellent sources for cholesterol which can aid in testosterone boosting. Blue cheese also has healthy bacteria and probiotics that can aid in testosterone elevation. Put them all together for maximum flavor and boost.

Yield: 4

Cooking Time:

List of Ingredients:

- Hamburger buns (4)
- Bacon (8 slices)
- Sea salt
- Red onion (½, sliced)
- Blue cheese (½ cup)
- Mayonnaise (1 cup)
- Beef (1 ½ lbs., ground)
- Dijon mustard (4 tbsp.)
- Black pepper
- Mushrooms (4, white mushrooms, sliced)
- Cheddar cheese (4 slices)

- Lettuce

sssssssssssssssssssssssssssssssssssssssssssssssssss

Procedure:

1. Heat grill.

2. Combine beef with pepper, salt and mustard and form into 4 patties. Place on grill and cook for 5 minutes on each side then add cheddar slice and cook for 1 minute more.

3. Place onion, mushroom and bacon onto grill and cook until golden all over.

4. Slice buns and toast then layer as desired.

5. Serve and enjoy!

14) Turkey Tenderloins

No need to cook a whole turkey to gain their testosterone boosting qualities. These juicy tenderloins are filled with proteins that have a positive reaction on testosterone.

Yield: 4

Cooking Time: 25 minutes (excluding marinating time)

List of Ingredients:

- Turkey tenderloins (1 lb.)
- Dijon mustard (1 tbsp.)
- Soy sauce (3 tbsp.)
- Rosemary (2 tsp., dried, crushed)

ssssssssssssssssssssssssssssssssssssssssssssssssssssssssss

Procedure:

1. Put tenderloins in a Ziploc bad and put aside.

2. Combine mustard, rosemary and soy sauce and pour into bag. Seal and shake to coat and place in refrigerator for 1-4 hours.

3. Set broiler on medium and take turkey from marinade and place on a baking sheet. Broil for 13 minutes and then turn over and cook for an extra 12 minutes.

4. Slice and serve with chutney of choice.

15) Blue Cheese Stuffed Mushrooms Wrapped in Bacon

All you need are 3 ingredients to create and awesome smack that will melt in your mouth. Each ingredient has testosterone boosting qualities.

Yield: 5

Cooking Time: 30 minutes

List of Ingredients:

- Bacon (10 slices)
- Blue cheese
- Mushrooms (10, white button, whole)

sssssssssssssssssssssssssssssssssssssssssssssssssssssss

Procedure:

1. Set oven to 350°F.

2. Remove stems and fill space with cheese.

3. Use a slice of bacon to wrap mushroom and use a toothpick to hold together.

4. Place on a baking sheet and bake for 20 minutes.

5. Serve and enjoy!

16) Honey Bean Salad

Beans are simply magical and have the highest level of zinc than other vegetables. The zinc in beans act just as that in red meat and are also high in protein. Kidney beans paired with a honey herb sauce, simply delicious!

Yield: 6

Cooking Time: 10 minutes

List of Ingredients:

- Canned kidney beans (10 oz.)
- Sage (1 tsp., dried)
- Honey (1 tbsp.)
- Canned Chickpeas (10 oz.)
- Garlic (2 cloves, diced)
- Apple cider vinegar (2 tbsp.)
- Hot sauce (1/8 tsp.)
- Canned Black beans (10 oz.)
- Black pepper (½ tsp.)
- Olive oil (2 tbsp.)
- Basil (1 tsp., dried)

- Red onion (1 sliced)

ssssssssssssssssssssssssssssssssssssssssssssssssssss

Procedure:

1. Drain beans and put into a bowl along with vinegar, onion, basil, hot sauce, olive oil, honey, black pepper, sage and garlic.

2. Stir to combine and serve!

17) Parmesan Spinach Cakes

Spinach contains magnesium which increases testosterone levels. These spinach cakes are great to grab to go and can be eaten for lunch or dinner.

Yield: 4

Cooking Time: 40 minutes

List of Ingredients:

- Spinach (12 oz.)
- Parmesan cheese (½ cup, grated)
- Garlic (1 clove, diced)
- Black pepper (¼ tsp.)
- Ricotta cheese (½ cup, part skim)
- Eggs (2, beaten)
- Salt (¼ tsp.)

ssssssssssssssssssssssssssssssssssssssssssssssssssss

Procedure:

1. Set oven to 400°F.

2. Put spinach into food processor and pulse until chopped then place into bowl along with eggs, salt, ricotta, garlic, pepper and Parmesan; mix to combine.

3. Grease muffin tin with cooking spray and spoon mixture into molds.

4. Bake for 20 minutes or until set. Remove from heat and cool in pan for 5 minutes.

5. Remove from pan and serve topped with Parmesan.

18) Broccoli with Garlic Butter and Cashews

This simple side is made with all testosterone boosting ingredients: garlic, broccoli and cashews. Crunchy and nutty with a hint of butter and can be paired with many lean meats.

Yield: 6

Cooking Time: 20 minutes

List of Ingredients:

- Broccoli (1 ½ lbs., chopped)
- White vinegar (2 tsp.)
- Butter (1/3 cup)
- Black pepper (¼ tsp.)
- Brown sugar (1 tbsp.)
- Garlic (2 cloves, diced)
- Soy sauce (3 tbsp.)
- Cashews (1/3 cup, salted and chopped)

SSSSSSSSSSSSSSSSSSSSSSSSSSSSSSSSSSSSSSSSSSSSSSSSSSSSSSS

Procedure:

1. Place an inch of water into a pot along with broccoli; cook for 7 minutes until tender. Drain and put aside on a platter until needed.

2. Heat skillet and melt butter then add soy sauce, pepper, sugar, garlic and vinegar and bring to a boil. Add cashews and pour over broccoli.

3. Serve and enjoy!

19) Creamy Spinach Dip

This creamy dip is healthy and can also be used as a spread. No easier way to boost that testosterone than with a dip. You can pair it with chips or veggies.

Yield: 4-6

Cooking Time: 10 minutes

List of Ingredients:

- Water Chestnuts (5 oz. can)
- Cottage cheese (½ cup, low fat)
- Yogurt (¼ cup, non-fat)
- Salt (½ tsp.)
- Baby spinach (6 oz.)
- Shallot (1, peeled)
- Cream cheese (½ cup, low fat)
- Lemon juice (1 tbsp.)
- Black pepper
- Chives (2 tbsp., chopped)

sssssssssssssssssssssssssssssssssssssssssssssssssssssss

Procedure:

1. Put chestnuts and shallot into processor and pulse until chopped then add cottage cheese, lemon juice, pepper, cream cheese, yogurt and salt and process until combined.

2. Add chives and spinach and blend to combine.

3. Serve and enjoy.

20) Broccoli and Brussels Sprout

Broccoli, Brussels sprout and other cruciferous vegetables are high in indoles which indirectly help boost testosterone. Indoles target estrogen and help decrease the amount in the body which give our 'T' count a chance to flourish.

Yield: 4

Cooking Time: 25 minutes

List of Ingredients:

- Butter (3 tbsp.)
- Tomato (1, seeds removed and minced)
- Garlic (2 cloves, diced)
- Salt (¼ tsp.)
- Broccoli florets (2 cups)
- Red pepper flakes (1/8 tsp.)
- Brussels sprouts (8, trimmed and cut in halves)

sssssssssssssssssssssssssssssssssssssssssssssssssssss

Procedure:

1. Heat skillet and melt a tbsp. of butter, add garlic and sauté for 1-2 minutes. Add sprouts and broccoli to garlic along with tomato and leftover butter. Add pepper flakes and salt to taste.

2. Cover pot and cook until golden and then turn over and cook for an additional 4 minutes.

21) Smoked Oyster Spread

All the ingredients used in this dish are ready made and combine for a filling dish. This can be made and refrigerated and used as much as you please.

Yield: 12

Cooking Time: 8 minutes

List of Ingredients:

- Canned oysters (1.7 oz., smoked)
- Worcestershire sauce (½ tsp.)
- Cream cheese (1.5 oz., soft)
- Lemon pepper

sssssssssssssssssssssssssssssssssssssssssssssssssssssssss

Procedure:

1. Use a fork to crush oysters in a bowl.

2. Add all leftover ingredients to oysters and stir to combine.

3. Chill and serve.

22) Brazilian Nut Berry Smoothie

Incorporating your Brazilian nuts into the start of your day will ensure you gain all the rewards it has to offer at the beginning of your day. You can use the nuts to create a 'milk' like base for your smoothies.

Yield: 2

Cooking Time: 30 minutes

List of Ingredients:

- Strawberries (1 cup)
- Blueberries (1 cup)
- Water (3 cups)
- Bananas (2, large)
- Flax seeds (2 tbsp., ground)
- Sea salt
- Raspberries (1 cup)
- Brazil nuts (2/3 cup, raw)
- Ice (½ cup)
- Prunes (1/8 cup, chopped, pits removed)
- Cinnamon (¼ tsp.)

sssssssssssssssssssssssssssssssssssssssssssssssssssss

Procedure:

1. Put all ingredients into blender and pulse until smooth.

2. Serve and enjoy!

23) Roasted Garlic Mashed Purple Potatoes

Thyme and roasted garlic infuse the mash potatoes for a herbed blend. Garlic contains a chemical called diallyl disulfide which promotes the release of a hormone that makes testosterone.

Yield: 10

Cooking Time: 60 minutes

List of Ingredients:

- Garlic (1 head)
- Thyme (1/3 oz.)
- Sour cream (½ cup, low fat)
- Salt (½ tsp.)
- Olive oil (¼ cup, extra-virgin)
- Potatoes (2lbs, purple/white, cubed)
- Milk (½ cup, low fat)
- Black pepper (¼ tsp.)

sssssssssssssssssssssssssssssssssssssssssssssssssssss

Procedure:

1. Set oven to 400°F.

2. Remove peel from garlic without separating cloves. Slice off the top to expose cloves. Put into a baking dish and add oil along with thyme. Cover pan with foil and bake for 30-45 minutes. Remove from heat, uncover and cool.

3. Prepare potatoes by boiling in salted water for 8-12 minutes until tender. Drain and put into a bowl.

4. Squeeze garlic out of shell and put with potatoes. Drizzle oil from garlic over potatoes and throw away thyme.

5. Add milk, black pepper, sour cream and salt; mash until thoroughly combined.

24) Buttery Brazil Nut Cookies

Brazilian nuts contain selenium which is also helpful in increasing testosterone levels. These nuts are delicious but be careful, one but contains 68-91 mcg and you have to try not to exceed 400 mcg. These cookies are made from only 5 ingredients.

Yield: 18

Cooking Time: 60 minutes

List of Ingredients:

- Brazil nuts (1 ¼ cups)
- Butter (¾ cup, salted)
- Vanilla (1 tsp.)
- Flour (2 cups)
- Confectioners' sugar (1 ¼ cups)

sssssssssssssssssssssssssssssssssssssssssssssssssssssss

Procedure:

1. Set oven to 325°F. Use parchment paper to line baking sheet and grease with cooking spray.

2. Put flour and nuts into processor and pulse until ground finely. Try not to over grind until oils come from nuts.

3. Put butter in a bowl and use mixer to beat then add vanilla and ¼ cup sugar and mix until combined. Add flour mixture and beat until a dough is formed. Mixture will look dry.

4. Form into balls and place onto lined sheet then bake for 25-30 minutes until slightly golden.

5. Put leftover sugar in a bowl and roll baked cookies in sugar right as they are taken from the oven.

6. Cool, serve and enjoy.

25) Roasted Garlic and Herb Bread

Use this garlicky bread to make a sandwich to start your day or even at lunch just remember to have a mint after. Your testosterone will thank you for this simple yet helpful aid.

Yield: 6 (12 slices)

Cooking Time: 2 ¼ hours

List of Ingredients:

- Garlic (2 heads, roasted)
- Flour (1 ¼ cups)
- Baking powder (1 tbsp.)
- Salt (½ tsp.)
- Eggs (2)
- Olive oil (1/3 cup, extra-virgin)
- White flour (1 ¼ cups, whole wheat)
- Fresh herbs (2 ¼ tbsp.)
- Baking sda (¼ tsp.)
- Black pepper (¼ tsp.)
- Milk (1 ¼ cups, low fat)

SSSSSSSSSSSSSSSSSSSSSSSSSSSSSSSSSSSSSSSSSSSSSSSSSSSSSS

Procedure:

1. Put rack in middle of oven and set to 375°F. Use parchment paper to line a loaf pan and use cooking spray to coat.

2. Remove peel from garlic and put cloves aside till needed.

3. Combine flours, baking powder, salt, 2 tbsp. herbs, black pepper and baking soda in a bowl using a whisk. Put oil, milk and eggs in another bowl and whisk to combine then add liquid mix to dry mix and combine then add cloves and fold. Put batter into prepared loaf pan and use spoon to smooth top. Use herbs to sprinkle over top.

4. Bake for 40-45 minutes. Remove from heat and cool for 15 minutes then remove from pan and cool for an extra 30 minutes.

5. Slice, serve and enjoy!

About the Author

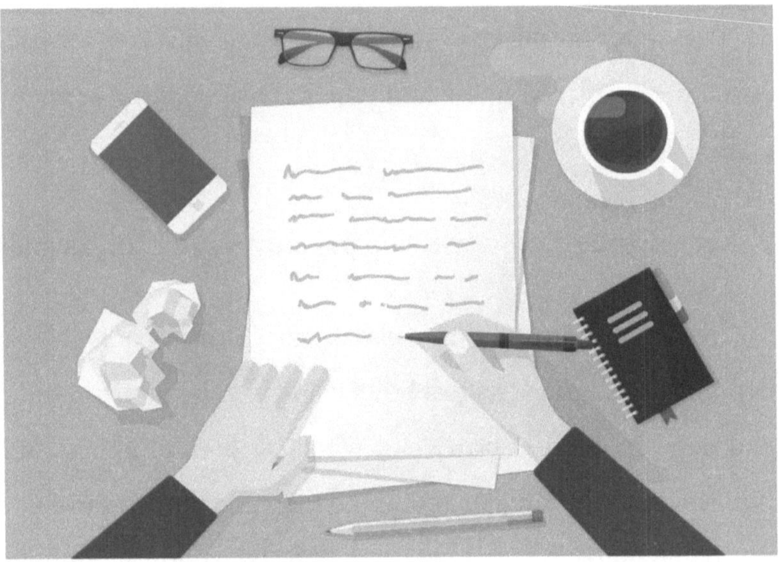

Allie Allen developed her passion for the culinary arts at the tender age of five when she would help her mother cook for their large family of 8. Even back then, her family knew this would be more than a hobby for the young Allie and when she graduated from high school, she applied to cooking school in London. It had always been a dream of the young chef to study with some of Europe's best and she made it happen by attending the Chef Academy of London.

After graduation, Allie decided to bring her skills back to North America and open up her own restaurant. After 10 successful years as head chef and owner, she decided to sell her business and pursue other career avenues. This monumental decision led Allie to her true calling, teaching. She also started to write e-books for her students to study at home for practice. She is now the proud author of several e-books and gives private and semi-private cooking lessons to a range of students at all levels of experience.

Stay tuned for more from this dynamic chef and teacher when she releases more informative e-books on cooking and baking in the near future. Her work is infused with stores and anecdotes you will love!

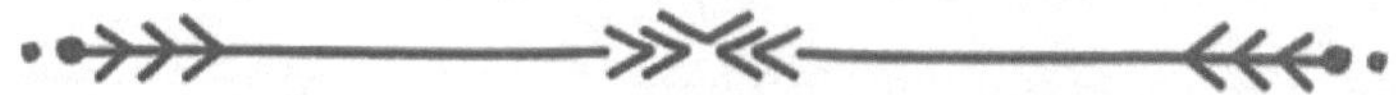

Author's Afterthoughts

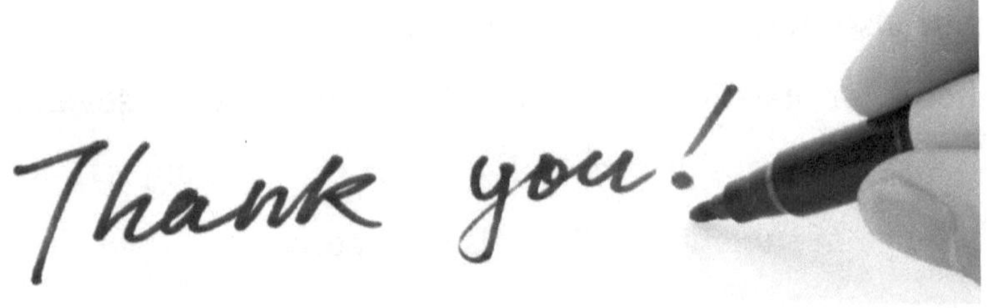

I can't tell you how grateful I am that you decided to read my book. My most heartfelt thanks that you took time out of your life to choose my work and I hope you find benefit within these pages.

There are so many books available today that offer similar content so that makes it even more humbling that you decided to buying mine.

Tell me what you thought! I am eager to hear your opinion and ideas on what you read as are others who are looking for a good book to buy. Leave a review on Amazon.com so others can benefit from your wisdom!

With much thanks,

Allie Allen